Nurse Heal Thyself
7 Strategies to Prevent Burnout & Maintain Positive Mental Health

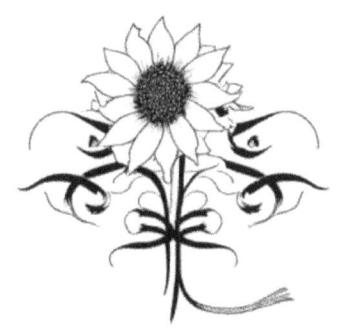

Tamara Sunflower

Nurse Heal Thyself

Copyright © 2023 Tamara Sunflower

Editing & Illustration Judith Z. Ulrich

All rights reserved. This book or any portion thereof may not be reproduced or used in any manner whatsoever without the express written permission of the publisher except for the use of brief quotations in a book review or scholarly journal.

ISBN: 9798341231009

Imprint: Independently published

First Printing: 2024

lajeunern@yahoo.com

With the assistance of https://kdp.amazon.com

Printed in the United States of America

Dedication

This book is dedicated to my earthly mother, Helen Melton, and father, Garling Lamon Theus. Without you, I wouldn't be here on planet Earth—much love and gratitude to God, Universe, and all my family and friends.

Acknowledgment

I have many supporters of my dreams and visions. I want to thank my dear husband, Philip McGoldrick, who has supported every dream, my sons, Demetre Theus and Christopher McGoldrick.

To all my family of sisters, brothers, aunts, uncles, cousins, nieces, nephews, grandchildren, and great grandchildren.

To all the McGoldrick family members all over the world.

Special thanks to Judy Ulrich for editing & illustration to make my dreams come true.

Warm fuzzies to all my friends and coworkers who shared this journey with me.

This book was inspired by my mother's best friend, Helen Bennett. She would come to our house, meet with my mother, and tell the most amazing nursing stories. She would wear her all-white uniform with the funny hat on her head. My mother would fix her a morning meal and drink coffee. I was about nine years old. I would hug the living room walls with my ears to listen in on her amazing stories that struck up excitement in my curious young mind.

I was taught to respect grown folks' conversations, so I did my best to listen intently from behind the living room wall. I knew then in my heart that I desired to become a nurse one day.

About the Author

Tamara Sunflower is a Native American Creek Indian (Muscogee Creek Tribe) who resides between Tulsa, Oklahoma and Salinas, California.

Tamara was raised in Southern California. She is mother, grandmother, great grandmother, author, entrepreneur, educator, and retired registered nurse with over forty years of experience in servicing children, adolescents, and adults with severe mental illness. She's a life coach for nurses.

Preface

With *Nurse Heal Thyself – 7 Strategies to Prevent Burnout & Maintain Positive Mental Health*, you will embark on a journey of discovery, resilience, and self-care specifically tailored to nurses. Nurses face unique challenges as caregivers that demand physical, emotional, and mental fortitude.

The demanding nature of the profession often takes a toll on their well-being, leading to burnout and potentially negative consequences for both the nurse and the patients they care for.

This preface serves as an invitation to explore the upcoming book, where we will delve into the depths of preventing burnout and maintaining positive mental health as a nurse. It is a heartfelt offering born out of a deep appreciation and admiration for the nursing profession and a genuine desire to support nurses in their pursuit of well-being.

You will find valuable insights, practical strategies, actionable tools to help you navigate the challenges that arise in the nursing profession. This book is not a mere collection of theoretical concepts or empty platitudes; it is a comprehensive guide infused with empathy, understanding, and real-life experiences.

While drawing upon the wisdom of healthcare professionals, mental health experts, and nurses, a roadmap has been crafted to help you prioritize your well-being, build resilience, and create a sustainable and fulfilling career in nursing. Each chapter addresses specific aspects of preventing burnout, offering practical strategies to implement in your daily life.

As you immerse yourself in these pages, you will discover the importance of self-care, the power of mindfulness, the significance of work-life balance, and the impact of positive thinking.

You will explore the vital role of effective communication and building strong relationships with colleagues and leaders. Moreover, you will gain insights into recognizing the signs of burnout and knowing when to seek help while advocating for healthy workplace environments and positive change.

Our hope is that this book serves as a trusted companion, offering solace, guidance, and encouragement whenever you need it most. We acknowledge the immense dedication and resilience you bring to your role as a nurse, and we believe that by investing in your own well-being, you can continue to provide exceptional care to those who depend on you.

It is our privilege to walk alongside you on this journey of self-discovery, and growth. Let us embark on this path together, supporting one another and creating a community that values and nurtures the mental health of nurses.

May this book be a source of inspiration, transformation and a wellspring of knowledge, and a catalyst for positive change as you navigate the noble path of nursing.

Contents

Dedication i
Acknowledgment ii
About the Author iii
Preface iv
Introduction 1
Chapter 1: Understanding Burnout Symptoms and Negative Effects of Stress That Leads to Burnout in Nurses, Causes of Burnout Among Nurses 7
Chapter 2: Time Management Aids in Preventing Stress and Burnout in Your Nursing Career, and Daily Routine 19
Chapter 3: Self-Care Practices 25
Chapter 4: Healthy Work-Life Balance . 31
Chapter 5: Building a Support System ... 37
Chapter 6: Positive Thinking 41
Chapter 7: Seeking Professional Help 47
Bonus Chapter 55
Notes 69

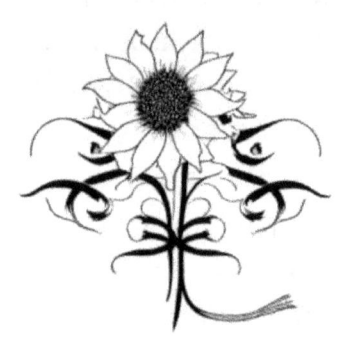

Introduction

As caregivers, nurses experience abundant stress and emotional exhaustion, often leading to burnout. Preventing burnout is essential to maintain your mental health, which eventually contributes to increased job satisfaction, improved patient care, and decreased turnover rates.

In this book, you will explore methods to prevent burnout for nurses to improve their overall physical and mental well-being, providing strategies to cope with stressful situations and promoting a positive work environment.

Ranging from self-care methods to mindfulness practices, each chapter focuses on a unique aspect of preventing and managing burnout for those who work as nurses.

With the implementation of these strategies, nurses can heal on a personal level and cultivate a fulfilling career in healthcare while providing top-notch care for their patients. Nurses also need to feel job satisfaction as well as a valued employee. The fact is, nursing is a very demanding career, and somebody has to do it.

I wrote this book with you in mind, to inspire, educate and share the importance of understanding the impact stress and burnout can have on your well-being and nursing career.

My desire is to express heartfelt gratitude to every nurse because what you do is very important to healthcare and helping patients get better. Nurses are on the frontline. You see things nobody else sees and advocate for the healing patient to get well.

As you carry on reading the book, you may embrace a sense of empowerment and understanding of how important your role is as a caring nurse and team player to administer excellent patient care.

I intend that as you read this book and identify with your personal experiences in your field of nursing, you can use these strategies shared in this book to accelerate your self-awareness and manage your life in such a way that is balanced, rewarding, and leads you to have a long-lasting career in nursing.

You may also find these strategies will help you heal by looking after yourself, managing stress, and preventing burnout.

This book is divided into seven chapters, each providing practical information to prevent and manage nurse burnout. Chapter 1 explores the need for understanding burnout, dives into the causes of burnout in nurses, and describes the negative effects stress can have on nurses.

Chapter 2 identifies and recognizes the importance of time management and prioritizing daily routines. Chapter 3 explores the concept of self-care and its importance in preventing burnout, offering ways to prioritize personal well-being, and introducing you to the benefits of mindfulness, explaining how the practice can aid in reducing stress levels and enhancing focus.

Chapter 4 helps nurses to understand the need for a healthy work-life balance, the importance of work-life balance in preventing burnout, and tips for managing work and personal life.

Chapter 5 emphasizes the importance of developing strong relationships with colleagues and leaders to promote a positive work environment while examining how impactful communication can reduce burnout and improve job satisfaction.

Chapter 6 explores the power of positive thinking and discovering techniques for training your mind to think positively. It also sheds light on processing the impact of trauma and how nurses can cope with its emotional toll.

Finally, Chapter 7 reflects on the importance of seeking help, strategies for accessing and utilizing mental health resources, and when to seek help for burnout and mental health issues. In addition to that, it also discusses the subjects of promoting healthy workplace environments and advocating for change.

Surely, *Nurse Heal Thyself* will be transformative for the rest of your life as you embrace the recommended strategies.

NURSE HEAL THYSELF

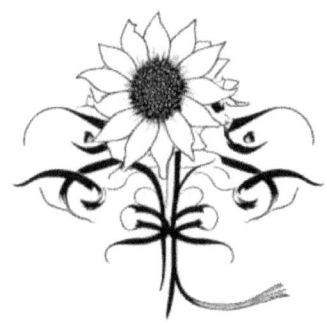

"As a nurse, we have the opportunity to heal the heart, mind, soul, and body of our patients, their families and ourselves. They may forget your name, but they will never forget how you made them feel."

– Maya Angelou

Chapter 1: Understanding Burnout Symptoms and Negative Effects of Stress That Leads to Burnout in Nurses, Causes of Burnout Among Nurses

Stress is a psychological or emotional response to an event or situation that is perceived as challenging or threatening. Various factors, including work, personal relationships, financial issues, and health problems, can cause it. However, the impact of stress can manifest itself in several ways, as evident through physical symptoms.

Let's dive deeper into understanding the ways stress, whether acute or chronic stress, can manifest in our bodies and impact our lives if not identified and managed.

Many factors impact a nurse's life that leads to burnout, such as unexpected deaths, working for long hours when staffing shortages need coverage, marriage, and relationship difficulties, having multiple stressors on the job and family life, and unresolved conflict.

Other than that, multiple issues like untreated depression and anxiety, poor self-esteem, traumatic and unexpected crises in one's life, not feeling valued at your job, substance abuse and illicit drug use, and many more can also affect the well-being of a nurse.

Unidentified stress can also pile up and leave a nurse feeling hopeless and helpless, which can affect the daily performance on the job, including missed workdays, showing up late, or creating many mistakes in your everyday working practices that can surely take a toll on you and your staff. All of these occurrences can lead to burnout and mental breakdown if unrecognized. The negative stressors can eventually lead to health concerns and possibly losing one's job.

Understanding the mechanics of stress is vital for every nurse because what's stressful to one nurse may not be stressful to another nurse. You have a level of coping with stressors, and how you manage stress as it presents to you personally is important to recognize and understand.

There are two kinds of stress. First, there is acute stress: short-term stress generally goes away quickly. Some examples are identified as feeling when you slam on the brakes while driving your car, having a fight with your partner, or skiing down a steep slope. Other examples of acute stress are preparing for a new job or becoming a new mother.

Acute stress symptoms can share the same characteristics as (PTSD) Post Traumatic Stress Disorder. The main difference is the duration of the symptoms, which can include:

- Faster heartbeat and rate
- Increased perspiration
- Increased irritability
- Having no memory of a traumatic event
- Avoiding people, places, or things that remind you of the traumatic event
- Hyperarousal, focus
- Feeling numb and detached, having reduced awareness of surroundings
- Feeling restless or being easily startled
- Having distressing thoughts, dreams, nightmares, and flashbacks of the event
- Having difficulty focusing your attention
- Feeling tense
- Feeling heightened irritability, sometimes leading to disgust or hatred of others

Secondly, chronic stress is defined as ongoing and consistent stress with no end or relief in sight. It can be very common for people dealing with prolonged health issues or disabilities or those who are looking after someone with prolonged health issues or disabilities.

Chronic stress can be seen in people who are dealing with longer-term situations, such as living with an abusive spouse, and high-stress and dangerous jobs, such as firefighters and police officers. Never taking a vacation or a break can surely lead to burnout.

Besides that, it can concern emergency medical workers such as nurses, doctors, medical paramedics, armed forces or military service men and women, crisis response teams, disaster prepared workers, ongoing housing, and financial difficulties, living in high-crime cities or neighborhoods. It can also impact anyone experiencing discrimination based on gender, sexual orientation, race, age, disability, religion, cultural background, etc.

The issue can also affect individuals with low self-esteem, someone dealing with multiple stressors at the same time, and mental health issues with limited support systems in place, such as friends and family.

Chronic stress over time can take a toll on your mental and physical health. Stress hormones called Cortisol are released to help your mind and body deal with a difficult situation and continue to be released due to prolonged ongoing stress.

As a result, the constant blood flow overload of hormones builds up over time and causes significant damage to our bodies. Signs and symptoms of Chronic Stress include the following:

- Memory problems and poor recall

- Poor decision making
- Nausea and digestive problems
- Overeating and weight gain or weight loss
- Depression, anxiety, and irritability
- Low self-esteem
- Substance abuse of any kind, alcohol & illicit drugs
- Addictive gambling, overspending
- Insomnia and fatigue
- High blood pressure
- Cardiovascular disease
- Headaches
- Reproductive concerns and low sex drive
- Poor concentration
- Type 2 Diabetes
- Increased risk of stroke or heart attacks

Keep in mind the first way to heal yourself is through gaining a sound knowledge of self-awareness. Listen to your body and know if you are experiencing any of the symptoms mentioned above, you must be proactive in looking at your life and be honest with yourself.

I have learned through my own personal life as a mental health nurse that I had to stop and realize what stressors I had in my own life while trying to provide excellent care for others.

I put my problems on the back burner until the walls came crashing down one day. I was working in the community as a registered nurse case manager for Veterans Affairs, and the stressors of driving one hour and a half one way daily in traffic to and from work were only one stress factor since I also had to organize my day to help my Veterans to manage their own lives.

Over time the stress can lead to burnout and health concerns. I was also helping my brother care for my elderly mother. I managed well until 2020 when the pandemic hit.

Unfortunately, I contracted Covid in May 2022, and symptoms of poor memory and poor concentration, no taste or smell, and being unable to continue with my position. I was forced to retire since my nursing license expired as well.

Thoughts of suicide entered my mind when my life came to that dead-end crossroads. I always had a spiritual relationship with God and had come to Jesus' visitation to find my way back into a place of serenity. Only God could save me with many prayers and soul-searching to heal my mind, body, and soul.

I had to do something to help myself. One of the questions I asked myself was, who will save me? However, using the strategies I mention in this book helped me sustain my nursing career for over thirty years.

Easy to use

The Perceived Stress Scale is easy to use and administer. You can quickly complete this test, gaining valuable insights time-efficiently.

First, identify that you are stressed and what you can do to reduce it. I have provided this tool for your use. The Perceived Stress Scale is provided below to measure your current stress level. It's an easy and dependable resource to measure your stress level.

Secondly, it is important to manage stress with the help of relaxation techniques, exercise, healthy eating, and seeking support from friends and family or professional help if necessary.

The importance of self-awareness is vital for every nurse in preventing burnout. Let's identify your stressors by utilizing this stress tool, the Perceived Stress Scale.

Accurate Results

The Perceived Stress Scale is a validated measure of perceived stress, so you can expect the results to be accurate and reliable.

This tool used to measure stress is the Perceived Stress Scale (PSS), a classic stress instrument developed in 1983, and it remains popular even today for helping you understand how different situations affect our feelings and our perceived stress.

Use the PSS score range to determine your level of stress.

You can determine your level of stress by using the PSS score range. If your total score is between 0 and 13, you are under stress. Scores between 14 and 26 indicate moderate stress, while scores between 27 and 40 indicate high perceived stress. For each question choose from the following alternatives.

The Perceived Stress Scale is a validated measure of perceived stress, so you can expect the results to be accurate and reliable.

This tool used to measure stress is the Perceived Stress Scale (PSS), a classic stress instrument developed in 1983, and it remains popular even today for helping you understand how different situations affect our feelings and our perceived stress.

Use the PSS score range to determine your level of stress.

You can determine your level of stress by using the PSS score range. If your total score is between 0 and 13, you are under stress. Scores between 14 and 26 indicate moderate stress, while scores between 27 and 40 indicate high perceived stress. For each question below choose from the following alternatives.

0-Never, 1-Almost Never, 2- Sometimes, 3- Fairly Often, 4- Very Often

1. In the last month, how often have you been upset because of something that happened unexpectedly?
2. In the last month, how often have you felt that you were unable to control the important things in your life?
3. In the last month, how often have you felt nervous and stressed?
4. In the last month, how often have you felt confident about your ability to handle your personal problems?
5. In the last month, how often have you felt that things were going your way?
6. In the last month, how often have you found that you could not cope with all the things that you had to do?

7. In the last month, how often have you been able to control irritations in your life?

8. In the last month, how often have you felt that you were on top of things?

9. In the last month, how often have you been angered because of things that happened outside your control?

10. In the last month, how often have you felt difficulties were piling up so high that you could not overcome them?

Figuring Your PSS Score

You can determine your PSS score by following these directions:

• First, reverse your scores for questions 4, 5, 7, and 8. On these four questions, change the scores like this:

0 = 4, 1 = 3, 2 = 2, 3 = 1, 4 = 0.

Now add up your scores for each item to get a total. My total score is _____.

• Individual scores on the PSS can range from 0 to 40, with higher scores indicating higher perceived

Use the PSS score range to determine your level of stress.

You can determine your level of stress by using the PSS score range. You are under stress if your total score is between 0 and 13. Scores between 14 and 26 indicate moderate stress, while scores between 27 and 40 indicate high perceived stress.

It is important to remember that the PSS is not a diagnostic tool, and if you have any additional concerns about your current state of health, you should seek medical attention.

The Perceived Stress Scale is an excellent tool for gaining insight into your current stress level and identifying areas where you need to focus on reducing stress in your life.

It is critical to use the test as a guide, not as a replacement for professional advice. If your stress levels are high, you must seek help from a mental health professional.

> *"Education is the most powerful weapon which you can use to change the world."*
>
> **– Nelson Mandela**

Chapter 2: Time Management Aids in Preventing Stress and Burnout in Your Nursing Career, and Daily Routine

Prioritizing nursing duties and managing time effectively at the same time are essential skills for nurses to maintain a balance between their personal lives and demanding careers.

Here are some strategies to help prioritize tasks and manage time effectively. I used these to help my nursing career stay organized, prioritize, and manage my time effectively. You can choose what works best for you since everyone operates differently.

1. Clear Goals

Determine short- and long-term goals for personal and professional life and prioritize tasks accordingly. Focus on being realistic about what can be achieved within a given time frame.

It is best to focus on one goal at a time to achieve it effectively. Put all your energy into your goal - write it, visualize it, and activate it with emotions daily, and you will succeed and see your results.

2. Organize Tasks

Create a list of tasks that need to be completed and categorize them based on their urgency and importance using the Eisenhower Matrix. This matrix organizes tasks into four categories:

- Urgent and important
- Important but not urgent
- Urgent but not important
- Neither urgent nor important

3. Do What Makes You Happy in Life

It might seem too simplistic, but it's important to acknowledge and realize that your happiness and wellness are as important as your duties as a nurse.

4. Delegate Tasks

Assess which tasks can be delegated to others to make more time for priority tasks. Also, clearly communicate what needs to be done and provide necessary resources for successful completion.

5. Develop A Schedule

Establish a daily, weekly, and monthly schedule, allocating time for tasks in each category. Include time for self-care, personal life, break, and tasks specific to work.

6. Set Specific Deadlines

Assign deadlines for tasks and break bigger tasks into smaller steps with their deadlines. Smaller steps lead to bigger accomplishments. Monitor progress regularly to ensure that tasks are completed on schedule.

7. Limit Multitasking

Focus on one task at a time, as multitasking can increase the likelihood of mistakes and decrease efficiency. Try to complete tasks one by one in order of priority.

8. Organize Workspace

Keep essential work tools and documents organized and easily accessible as well. An orderly workspace can reduce distractions and cater to efficient task completion. De-clutter any surrounding workspace that needs to be sorted.

9. Avoid Procrastination

Recognize when procrastination occurs, and utilize strategies to overcome it, such as setting a timer for focused work or rewarding oneself after completing a task.

10. Be Adaptable

Review the priority list throughout the day and be prepared to adjust it when unforeseen circumstances are encountered. Be flexible in reallocating time for tasks when necessary.

With the help of implementing these steps, nurses can prioritize their nursing duties, manage time efficiently, and create a better balance between work and personal life. These strategic tools can effectively help improve time management by prioritizing your life.

Trust me, if you implement these strategies, your life will change, and you will find much-needed satisfaction. It will make your life more fulfilling, accompanied by satisfaction.

You can heal yourself by reducing stress and creating a better workflow and organized space leads to self-empowerment and fulfillment. You will experience more confidence and enjoy what you do as a nurse. A positive outcome will give you more energy to help with patient care and offer satisfaction working with your staff.

NURSE HEAL THYSELF

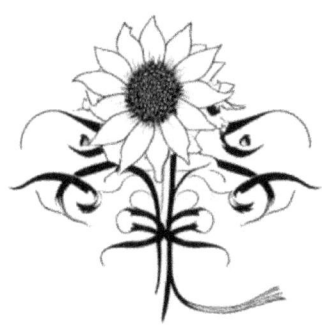

"Take care of your body. It's the only place you have to live."

– Jim Rohn

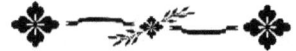

Chapter 3: Self-Care Practices

Strategies for Maintaining Mental Health

Identifying and Implementing Self-Care Practices that Work for You

Self-care promotes happiness and can be achieved through various practices and habits. Here is a list of methods I used personally to help improve my overall happiness and self-care practices:

Strategies

1. **Practice gratitude:** Regularly reflecting on what you are thankful for can foster a positive mindset and a greater sense of contentment. Choosing to write in a journal daily will keep cluttering thoughts out of your head and onto paper- ultimately, giving you more head space allows mental clarity is vital. There is power in Gratitude!

2. **Nurture relationships:** Building and maintaining strong relationships with friends, family, and colleagues can lead to emotional support and a sense of belonging.

We all need each other in some way. Nurses are usually caring and giving of themselves. It feels good when your coworker has your back in times of need. Teamwork is dream work, so reach out to your peers for additional support.

3. **Exercise regularly:** Physical activity has been proven to release endorphins and boost mood while improving overall physical health. If your schedule is busy, finding time to take a 15-minute walk or get off the unit is important for refreshing your mind and body. Take the staircase whenever possible instead of elevator if you are going a few floors up or down.

4. **Get adequate sleep:** Maintain a regular sleep schedule and prioritize getting enough rest to ensure physical and mental well-being. Sleep is very important for many reasons. Your body needs time to heal itself and to recharge your brain cells. I have always had insomnia and found useful ways to combat it since I worked the graveyard shift for much of my nursing career. A good night's sleep is vital for your healing and rejuvenation.

5. **Eat a balanced diet:** A healthy diet can promote overall health and contribute to mood stability, energy levels, and general happiness. Prepare your snacks and lunch ahead of time. I encourage you to keep healthy finger foods in your lunch bag, such as raw vegetables, separately or with salad dressing, and apple slices with peanut butter. However, if you are allergic, try almond butter: cheese, and crackers.

6. **Practice mindfulness and meditation:** Mindfulness can help reduce stress, improve focus, and enhance overall well-being. A great app to use is *Moonly* - this application is fantastic and cost-

efficient. This app combines mindfulness, astrology, and psychology. Include meditation applications and your astrological daily forecast for those who are conscious. Daily positive affirmations are included as well. I use it daily, and it helps to promote sleep and effective mindfulness. Choose an app that works for you there are many available

7. **Develop hobbies and interests:** Pursue activities you are passionate about to boost self-esteem, meet new people, and add variety to your life.

8. **Set and achieve goals:** Establish realistic and attainable goals that align with your values and celebrate your achievements. Even if the smallest wins, you should give yourself a pat and reward yourself.

Go get a pedicure or manicure. Buy your favorite ice cream, or purchase a new purse, clothing, or jewelry. I love rocky road ice cream from the local ice cream store, and I would get myself a double dip of pistachio nut and rocky road, and it felt like heaven on earth. I would lick it until I was so satisfied in my mouth down to my tummy. Sometimes I would pull over in my car after working a busy week and treat myself.

9. **Help others:** Engaging in acts of kindness and volunteering can generate feelings of accomplishment, satisfaction, and improved self-worth.

Find something you can do off duty to make a difference in someone's life. I would volunteer at the local food pantry and help sort the donated cans. You can pick up trash in your community or help serve lunch or dinner at the local Salvation Army. Donate a bag of clothing items you haven't worn in over a year or outgrown.

10. **Laugh and have fun:** Laughter can reduce stress hormones, increase feel-good endorphins, and help build social connections. Laughter is like medicine; you have heard that before. Use humor in good taste to make others laugh with you.

11. **Cultivate optimism:** Practice looking at situations positively and finding the bright side in challenging circumstances. Turn your negative situations into positive ones. For every negative thought replace it with three positive statements. Think out of the box by tapping into your intuition. Be creative.

12. **Learn to manage stress:** Develop healthy coping strategies for dealing with stress, such as deep breathing, yoga, or journaling. Say positive affirmations daily—generally, first thing in the morning and just before bed. Take a nice warm bath, include sea salt, and add lavender scent, bubble bath, and Epsom salts to promote healing in your body. Magnesium is very healing and relaxes your muscles.

13. **Foster self-compassion:** Practice being kind and understanding towards yourself during times of failure or difficulty. Use your failures as a learning experience. Ask yourself, what could I have done to improve the situation? You are born with unique and special traits. Embrace them. Be an original and not a follower. Use your creative mind to create a better work environment.

14. **Connect with nature:** Spending time outdoors can reduce stress, increase creativity, and promote happiness. Sitting in the sun for 10-15 minutes, walking on grass barefoot or sitting on the beach if you live near one, hugging a tree, or planting a garden can elevate your happiness. Take a walk in the park and listen to the sounds of nature.

15. **Limit comparisons:** Comparing yourself to others can be detrimental to your happiness. Focus on individual growth and accept yourself for who you are. You are made beautifully. Learn to embrace any flaws you think you have. You are a winner because you exist; remember, there is only one you. Clap your hands and reward yourself often. Sometimes we must be our own cheerleaders in life.

By incorporating these strategies into your daily life, you can actively work towards enhancing your happiness and promoting overall well-being so that you stay healthy and well.

> "The only person you are destined to become is the person you decide to be."
>
> – Ralph Waldo Emerson, Father of American literature

Chapter 4: Healthy Work-Life Balance

The importance of work-life balance in preventing burnout

Strategies for managing work and personal life

Maintaining a healthy work-life balance is essential to prevent burnout for nurses. The importance of work-life balance for nurses cannot be emphasized enough, as it plays a critical role in preventing burnout and ensuring their overall well-being.

Nursing is a demanding profession that requires long hours, high levels of stress, and emotional investment in patient care. Striking a balance between work and personal life allows nurses to dedicate time to self-care, mental health, and maintaining relationships with friends and family, which help reduce stress and enhance resilience.

Achieving a balance between personal and professional responsibilities gives nurses a sense of control and satisfaction in both aspects of their lives, ultimately fostering overall happiness and well-being.

By prioritizing work-life balance, nurses can ensure they remain effective in their roles, fostering a healthier workplace environment, improving patient care, and maintaining their mental and emotional health in the long term.

Here are some strategies I personally adopted to help me in my nursing career. I found them very helpful and hope you can incorporate them into your daily life to help you manage your professional and personal life. Balancing work life is vital for nurses to establish equilibrium between your personal and professional lives:

Strategies

1. **Set boundaries:** Define clear boundaries between work and personal life. Avoid taking work home or engaging in work-related activities during personal time. Communicate these boundaries to colleagues and family members. Remember you have a choice to say "No" if you need personal space & time.

2. **Prioritize self-care:** Engage in regular self-care practices, such as exercise, healthy eating, and getting sufficient sleep. Make time for hobbies and interests outside of work. Do something fun often and embrace good humor.

3. **Create a daily routine:** Establish a consistent routine that incorporates time for work, personal life, and self-care. It will help create a sense of structure and enable a better balance.

4. **Learn to delegate:** Identify tasks that can be delegated at work or home to help reduce stress and create more time for priorities.

5. **Set realistic expectations:** Be realistic about what can be achieved at and outside work. Focus on accomplishing tasks efficiently without overextending yourself.

6. **Develop time management skills:** Improve time management by prioritizing tasks, setting deadlines, and utilizing tools such as to-do lists or calendars. Get up 30 minutes early and go to bed early if possible.

7. **Nurture relationships:** Dedicate time to maintaining and fostering relationships with friends, family members, and colleagues. Strong social connections can provide valuable emotional support.

8. **Schedule breaks:** Regular breaks during work hours can help avoid burnout. Designate time for relaxation, quick physical activity, or moments of mindfulness. Have 15-minute breaks and rejuvenate your mind. Make sure you step away from what you are doing to clear your mind and go to a quieter space. Relaxing music can also be a great help.

9. **Manage stress:** Develop healthy coping mechanisms for dealing with stress, such as meditation, deep breathing exercises, or journaling.

Take the stress test provided in this book to see where you stand.

10. Unplug from technology: Make a conscious effort to disconnect from electronic devices during personal time, which can help reduce stress and promote better work-life balance.

11. Remain flexible: Be prepared to adapt to changes and adjust your work-life balance when needed, whether for personal or professional reasons.

12. Seek support: Utilize support networks, such as friends, family, or professional counseling, to help manage the challenges of maintaining a healthy work-life balance.

With the help of these strategies, nurses can create a healthy work-life balance, which is crucial in preventing burnout and maintaining mental well-being. Know thyself so you can heal thyself. Know your limits. Don't take on more than you can handle. Nurses tend to be co-dependent and overload themselves.

Stop right there!

It's okay to say "No."

NURSE HEAL THYSELF

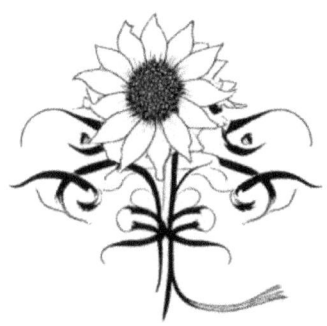

"If you want to lift yourself up, lift up someone else."

– **Booker T. Washington**

Chapter 5: Building a Support System

The benefits of having a support system

Strategies for building and maintaining a strong support system

Building a strong support system is essential in nursing to prevent burnout and maintain overall well-being. Here are five strategies to consider.

Firstly, consider actively networking and communicating with colleagues at work to foster camaraderie and teamwork. Sharing experiences and discussing challenges can create a support network within the workplace.

Secondly, seek mentorship from experienced nursing professionals who can provide guidance, encouragement, and a listening ear.

Thirdly, participate in peer support groups or professional team building organizations, both locally and online, to exchange ideas, share experiences, and gain valuable insights from other nurses.

Fourthly, nurture personal relationships with friends and family members, as they can help provide emotional support and an alternative perspective on work-related issues.

Lastly, consider seeking professional help from a therapist or mental health counselor to discuss experiences openly and develop coping mechanisms.

Remember, most jobs have an (EAP) -Employee Assistance Program. Use it if you need help; the information is kept discreetly to support you and your well-being.

A robust support system can help decrease burnout in nursing settings by providing emotional support, fostering feelings of belonging, encouraging problem-solving, and promoting overall resilience in the face of workplace challenges.

Maintaining strong connections can significantly reduce stressors' impact and promote a more positive work environment. I always say, "Cast a wide net." The more support you allow is to your benefit.

Strategies for building a strong support system are vital for nurses to offer support and team uplift. You are not alone and have a space to go when you need assistance, which helps reduce burnout and stress.

NURSE HEAL THYSELF

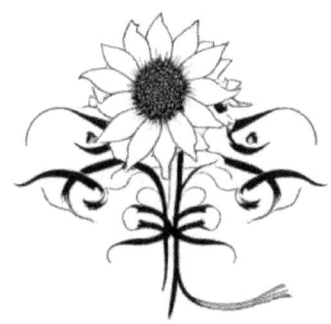

> *"**Expect the best.**
>
> *Convert problems into opportunities. Be dissatisfied with the status quo. Focus on where you want to go, instead of where you're coming from.*
>
> ***And most importantly, decide to be happy,** knowing it's an attitude, a habit gained from daily practice, and not a result or payoff."*
>
> – **Denis Waitley**

Chapter 6: Positive Thinking

The power of positive thinking

Techniques for training your mind to think positively

Adopting a positive mindset can have significant benefits in personal life and on the job as a nurse.

Firstly, thinking positively can lead to greater resilience and adaptability when facing challenges or setbacks, making coping with stress easier and staying focused on solutions rather than dwelling on problems. Shift your mindset for a favorable outcome.

Secondly, a positive outlook contributes to improved mental and physical health, as it has been associated with lower rates of anxiety and depression, better immune function, and increased longevity.

Thirdly, positive thinking can boost self-confidence and motivation, enabling nurses to overcome obstacles, learn from their experiences, and continue growing professionally.

Fourthly, maintaining a positive mindset can enhance interpersonal relationships with colleagues, patients, and family members, fostering empathy, understanding, and constructive communication.

Finally, embracing positivity contributes to a more enjoyable and fulfilling work environment, as it encourages a supportive and collaborative atmosphere, leading to increased job satisfaction and decreased burnout rates among nurses. Cultivating a positive outlook as a nurse can ultimately contribute to personal and professional success and overall well-being.

Strategies

Incorporating positive thinking into your daily life can benefit your mental health and overall well-being. Here are ten strategic techniques to help train your mind to think positively:

1. **Practice gratitude:** By regularly reflecting on things you are thankful for, fostering a mindset focused on abundance rather than scarcity. The gratitude journal is very helpful and healing. Journal as often as you need to get whatever is on your mind out of your head and onto paper. Release your energy to channel positively. Uncluttered mind space is priceless.

2. **Develop a personal mantra or affirmation:** By saying out loud daily- the daily mantra or affirmation reinforces positive beliefs about yourself, which can be repeated throughout the day. Scientific fact, saying something for 21 days can reset your thought pattern. See this book's "Bonus" section for suggestions of positive affirmations or develop your own.

3. **Surround yourself:** Interact with positive people who encourage, support, and uplift you; their attitudes can influence your mindset. Beware negative energy, and release yourself from toxic people, places, and things.

4. **Limit exposure:** Limiting negative media or content, opting for uplifting and inspirational material.

5. **Challenge negative thoughts:** By evaluating their accuracy, focusing on solutions, or replacing them with more optimistic perspectives. Try daily journaling and positive daily affirmations.

6. **Engage in activities**: Any activity that brings you joy, which can elicit positive emotions and improve your overall outlook. Be playful and allow yourself to be creative. Laugh out loud too!

7. **Visualization:** Visualization can be a powerful tool; imagine yourself in a positive situation or outcome, allowing your mind to absorb the positive feelings associated with that image. Practice mindfulness and meditation daily.

8. **Maintain a growth mindset:** Be flexible by viewing challenges and setbacks as opportunities to learn and improve rather than failures. Maintaining a flexible mind will help you from getting bogged down with stress.

9. **Implement acts of kindness:** Volunteer work and helping others can create satisfaction and happiness. Give something away. If you haven't worn certain clothing items in a year, consider supporting someone else. Donate them to local charities or someone you know who needs it. Local churches and food banks always need help.

10. **Practice mindfulness and meditation**: Get quiet to center your thoughts and cultivate an awareness of the present moment, training your mind to stay focused on the positive. There are many apps available like Moonly and Calm that can be assessable to you if downloaded to your phone.

Integrating these techniques into your daily routine allows you to gradually rewire your thought patterns and develop a more optimistic outlook on life.

NURSE HEAL THYSELF

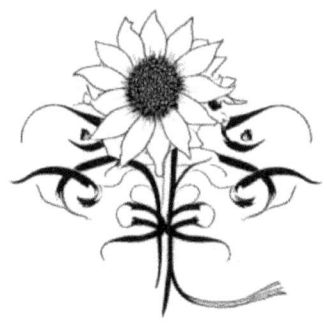

*"You're **braver** than you believe, **stronger** than you seem, and **smarter** than you think."*

- A.A. Milne Author Poet

Chapter 7: Seeking Professional Help

When seeking help for burnout and mental health issues, self-awareness is vital. You know yourself better than anyone else. Don't wait to ask for help.

Strategies For Accessing and Utilizing Mental Health Resources

Nurses must prioritize their mental health, especially given their high-stress work environment. There are several reasons why seeking help when mental health issues arise is essential:

1. **Protect personal well-being:** Addressing mental health challenges early can prevent long-term psychological distress, maintain overall well-being, and reduce the risk of developing severe mental health disorders.

2. **Preserve patient safety:** Nurses experiencing mental health struggles may have difficulty providing optimal care. By seeking help, nurses can ensure they maintain their ability to provide the best possible care for their patients.

From my experience of working with a team of nurses, I realized I couldn't do what I needed to do on my job and had to face the challenges of my health head-on since I couldn't perform and give my patients the best care possible. I cared enough for my patients; knowing I had to step away was best for me and my patients.

One day, I can remember driving in the governmental van. A veteran asked me if I was okay. I sheepishly said yes, realizing he noticed I wasn't myself. I haven't slept well for about a month or more, which showed in my physical appearance and work. So don't wait to get help when you know something is wrong with you. The first person that should know if something is wrong with you is you or those closest to you.

3. **Maintain job performance:** Unaddressed mental health issues may affect a nurse's performance, leading to decreased productivity, increased errors, and potential burnout. Seeking help can maintain job effectiveness and satisfaction.

4. **Set a positive example:** By prioritizing mental health and seeking help when needed, nurses can set an example for colleagues and create an open, supportive environment for discussing mental health concerns.

5. **Enhance coping skills:** Accessing mental health resources can empower nurses with strategies and tools to manage stress and difficult emotions, fostering increased resilience in the long term.

To assess and utilize mental health resources, consider the following strategies:

1. **Self-assess regularly:** Be mindful of your emotional and mental well-being. Monitor signs of distress, such as increased anxiety, irritability, or sleep disturbances, and act accordingly.

2. **Research available resources:** Familiarize yourself with mental health resources offered by your employer, such as Employee Assistance Programs (EAPs), peer support groups, or mental health professionals.

3. **Always seek professional help:** Consult a licensed therapist, psychologist, or psychiatrist for guidance and support.

4. **Engage in support groups:** Attend local or online support groups for healthcare professionals or nurses to share experiences and learn from others who have faced similar challenges.

5. **Leverage your social network:** Reach out to friends, family, and colleagues for support, as they may provide valuable insight, encouragement, and understanding. Keep all the important numbers on your phone.

Initially, it was difficult for me to ask for help. I finally reached out and found that help was available, and I felt so much better. The silverback gorilla was finally off my back.

Please, do yourself a favor and never be afraid to reach out to your supervisor to let them know you need help. Don't let it show up in your work performance. Healing thyself begins the moment you ask and seek help.

Promptly addressing mental health concerns is crucial for nurses to ensure their well-being, safety, and a thriving work environment. Here are some resources available to you:

National mental health organizations and crisis hotlines are vital in providing support, resources, and immediate assistance to individuals in need.

Some of these organizations include the National Alliance on Mental Illness (NAMI), which offers education, advocacy, and support for those affected by mental health conditions, and Mental Health America (MHA), which promotes mental wellness through advocacy, education, and support services.

One major observance during September is Suicide Prevention Awareness Month. The National Alliance on Mental Health (NAMI), said that we use this month to shift public perspective, spread hope, and share vital information. During the month of September, NAMI runs the "Together for Mental Health" campaign to encourage people to advocate for better mental health.

Additionally, the Substance Abuse and Mental Health Services Administration (SAMHSA) is a valuable resource for connecting individuals with appropriate mental health and substance abuse services.

In times of crisis or if you need immediate assistance, the National Suicide Prevention Lifeline offers 24/7 support through their toll-free hotline at 1-800-273-TALK (1-800-273-8255).

Another essential resource is the Crisis Text Line, which provides free, confidential help by texting "HELLO" to 741741. Besides that, you can also call 988, operated by Suicide and Crisis Lifeline. Both the hotline and the text line connect individuals with trained counselors who can provide aid, guidance, and support during a mental health crisis or emotional distress.

***

Throughout this book, I repeated some strategies simply because repeatedly reading them lets them sink into your mind. If you are stressed oftentimes, you don't retain information as well as you should. The goal is to heal thyself by choosing a clear sound mind and understanding your matter to the world, and using these strategies in this book will transform your life, decreasing stress and burnout. You can maintain positive mental health.

In closing, be sure to take your vacation if you have a week or two weeks. Even a three or four-day break is nice. Be sure to connect with nature as much as possible. Going for a simple walk for 15-30 minutes daily can be nice to revitalize your well-being.

Always remember you are needed in this world. Every day is a new day to heal you, change your mental thoughts to positive ones, and, most of all, heal your heart of any burdens. Everyone has a story to tell, and I encourage you to write a book. Let's stay connected. You can go to my email: lajeunern@yahoo.com.

Getting sunshine is so refreshing and good for your soul. Please protect your skin using sunscreen if you are exposed to direct sunlight for any length of time.

I do something called sun gazing early, about six o'clock am, and when the sun goes down in the evening. If you ever want to do sun gazing or moon gazing, that is looking into the sun or moon. Never do it mid-day when the sun is at its peak and brightest. It may cause damage to your eyes (retina). Also, always check in with your primary doctor before any physical activity. Check out the sun after it's going down in the evening. I do it no more than five or ten minutes at a time.

Please do your research on this technique before trying it. Please keep in mind this book is to be used as a source of support and guidance. It is not intended to diagnose or treat anyone medically.

NURSE HEAL THYSELF

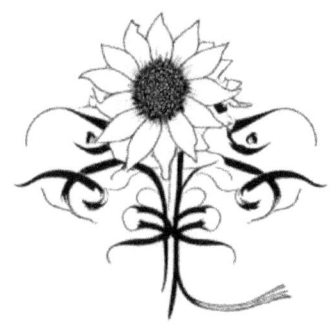

"There is no problem outside of you that is superior to the power within you."

-Bob Proctor

Bonus Chapter

Conscious Ways to Heal Thyself

You owe it to yourself to build paradise in your own home. You can always pay for a spa day if you choose. Getting full body massages once a month or every two months is a good way to relax. Pampering yourself is a must.

Even a good foot rub will foster healing in your feet. Either way, you work hard; you need to play even harder. Permitting yourself to self-care is vital to your inner healing as a nurse.

Have you heard the saying? "You cannot pour from an empty cup!" Pamper yourself as often as you feel you need it. I'm a big fan of aroma therapy and essential oils. My favorites are Lavender, Rose, and Patchouli.

Aromatherapy can help promote relaxation and alleviate stress. Here are five of the most relaxing essential oils often used in aromatherapy:

1. **Lavender:** Widely recognized for its calming properties, lavender essential oil is ideal for alleviating stress, anxiety, and insomnia. It is often used in bedtime routines to encourage a good night's sleep. Placing several drops on a cotton ball is a fun way to relax at work or home. Keep it nearby and

smell the cotton ball periodically to promote relaxation.

2. **Ylang-Ylang:** Known for its unique floral scent, ylang-ylang essential oil is especially soothing and can help reduce anxiety, stress, and tension. It also has uplifting properties that can promote positive emotions.

3. **Chamomile:** Roman chamomile essential oil possesses calming qualities that can help ease stress, anxiety, and irritability. Commonly used to promote relaxation in teas, chamomile oil is just as effective in aromatherapy.

4. **Bergamot:** This citrusy essential oil is derived from bergamot oranges and is known for reducing stress and anxiety. Bergamot has a balancing effect on the mind and emotions, promoting relaxation and renewal.

5. **Sandalwood:** Sandalwood essential oil, with its warm, woody scent, has grounding and calming properties that can help alleviate stress, anxiety, and mental fatigue. Its soothing fragrance is also known for encouraging deeper meditation and spiritual connection.

To utilize these essential oils in aromatherapy, consider diffusing them into the air, adding a few drops to a warm bath, or diluting them with a carrier oil to create a relaxing massage oil. Always follow proper safety guidelines for oil usage and dilution, as some essential oils can cause skin irritation if used undiluted.

Here are five recipes for making body salt scrubs using relaxing essential oils to promote relaxation:

1. Lavender and Patchouli Salt Scrub

- 1 cup Epsom salt or sea salt

- 1/2 cup sweet almond oil or coconut oil

- 15-20 drops of lavender essential oil and or same number of drops for Patchouli essential oil (optional)

- 1 tablespoon dried lavender flowers (optional)

Mix all ingredients, then store them in an airtight container.

2. Bergamot and Orange Salt Scrub

- 1 cup Epsom salt or sea salt

- 1/2 cup coconut oil or jojoba oil

- 10 drops of bergamot essential oil

- 10 drops of sweet orange essential oil

Combine all ingredients and mix well. Store the mixture in an airtight container.

3. Rose and Jasmine Salt Scrub

- 1 cup Epsom salt or sea salt

- 1/2 cup sweet almond oil or grapeseed oil

- 10 drops rose absolute oil

- 10 drops of jasmine essential oil

Mix all ingredients, then store the scrub in an airtight container.

4. Ylang-Ylang and Sandalwood Salt Scrub

- 1 cup Epsom salt or sea salt

- 1/2 cup fractionated coconut oil or sweet almond oil

- 10 drops of ylang-ylang essential oil

- 10 drops of sandalwood essential oil

Combine all ingredients and mix well. Transfer the scrub to an airtight container for storage.

5. Chamomile and Lavender Salt Scrub

- 1 cup Epsom salt or sea salt

- 1/2 cup olive oil or coconut oil

- 15 drops of lavender essential oil

- 5 drops Roman chamomile essential oil

Blend all ingredients and store the finished product in an airtight container.

To use these salt scrubs, gently massage a handful onto damp skin, avoiding sensitive areas, and rinse off with warm water. These relaxing body scrubs can help exfoliate and nourish the skin while providing a calming aromatherapeutic experience.

I love indoor plants. You may not have a green thumb but consider your environment to make yourself feel better. If you love plants, here are some good reasons to consider indoor plants and their benefits.

Indoor plants are visually appealing and can significantly benefit your health and well-being. They have the power to improve indoor air quality by reducing pollutants, such as volatile organic compounds (VOCs), carbon dioxide, and dust particles, which in turn can alleviate respiratory issues, allergies, and headaches.

Plants also contribute to humidity, maintaining a comfortable environment and reducing dry skin and irritation, and they also help relieve cold symptoms.

Additionally, the presence of plants has a positive effect on mental health, as they are known to reduce stress, elevate mood, and enhance concentration and productivity.

To create a healthier environment in your living space, consider incorporating these five indoor plants:

1. Spider Plant (Chlorophytum Comosum), an excellent air purifier and an easy-to-care plant
2. Snake Plant (Sansevieria trifasciata) is efficient at removing toxins and producing oxygen at night, making it suitable for bedrooms.
3. Peace Lily (Spathiphyllum spp), a beautiful plant with air-purifying abilities.
4. English Ivy (Hedera helix), adept at removing mold spores and other allergens.
5. Golden Pothos (Epipremnum aureum), a hardy plant that filters pollutants and enhances humidity. Incorporating these plants into your indoor space will invite various health benefits and foster a more comfortable living environment.

Daily Positive Affirmations

Positive self-love affirmations can help reinforce your self-worth, boost confidence, and encourage self-acceptance. Here are ten examples of self-love affirmations:

1. **Today**, I am worthy of love, happiness, and success. (Feel it, see it, and believe it)
2. **Today**, I embrace my unique qualities and appreciate my true self.

3. **Today,** I am confident in my abilities and believe in myself.

4. **Today,** I deserve the best in life and am open to receiving it.

5. **Today,** I love and respect my body and treat it with care and kindness.

6. **Today,** I trust my inner wisdom and intuition, allowing them to guide me.

7. **Today,** I choose to overcome any challenges and learn from them.

8. **Today,** I love my self-worth. It's not dependent on others' opinions; I know my value.

9. **Today,** I fill my mind with positive thoughts and focus on my strengths.

10. **Today,** I am constantly growing, evolving, and becoming the best version of myself.

Repeating these affirmations daily can gradually help rewire your thoughts and promote a healthier relationship with yourself, fostering a sense of self-love and acceptance.

I would like to recommend saying these out loud with your voice recording on your phone. Hearing your voice goes right to your subconscious mind. I do this first thing in the morning and just before bed.

Sleep Hygiene

Establishing a bedtime routine and enhancing sleep quality is vital for promoting physical and mental healing. Here are five tips for getting a good night's sleep:

1. **Create a consistent sleep schedule:** Going to bed and waking up at the same time daily helps regulate your internal clock, making it easier to fall asleep and wake up feeling refreshed. Balance yourself with a consistent sleep schedule.

2. **Develop a pre-sleep routine:** Engaging in calming activities before bedtime, such as reading, taking a warm bath, or practicing relaxation techniques, can signal to your body and mind that it's time to unwind and prepare for sleep.

3. **Limit exposure to screens:** Reducing screen time before bed, particularly blue light-emitting devices, can help prevent disruptions to your natural sleep cycle by decreasing the stimulation of brain activity and promoting the production of melatonin.

4. **Create a comfortable sleep environment:** Investing in a quality mattress and pillows, adjusting room temperature, reducing noise, and maintaining a dark bedroom are all essential to crafting a comfortable and conducive environment for pleasant sleep. Silence your phone and devices prior to

bedtime. Some people like the noise of a fan going can be relaxing and circulate air in the room.

5. **Avoid stimulants and heavy meals:** Reduce caffeine and nicotine consumption during the evening and avoid consuming heavy meals too close to bedtime. These substances and large meals can cause discomfort and interfere with your ability to fall asleep.

A bedtime routine is crucial for promoting healing, as quality sleep provides numerous benefits, including physical repair and restoration. While you sleep, your body focuses on healing damaged tissues, building bone and muscle, and generating hormones crucial for healthy functioning.

Moreover, adequate sleep is essential for optimal cognitive functioning, emotional regulation, and stress reduction, contributing to overall mental health and well-being.

Establishing a consistent bedtime routine and prioritizing sleep promotes physical, mental, and emotional healing that enables you to lead a healthier, more balanced life.

Creating A Personal Action Wellness Plan

A daily personal action wellness plan can be a valuable tool for taking charge of your self-care, ensuring that your physical, emotional, and mental well-being are prioritized throughout the month.

To successfully implement a self-care calendar for 31 days, identify key focus areas, such as exercise, nutrition, sleep, stress reduction, and social connections.

Next, assign specific activities or goals to each day, ensuring they are attainable and enjoyable for sustained motivation. For example, Mondays could be devoted to a 30-minute yoga session and a healthy and nutritious breakfast.

Tuesdays might involve journaling for 20 minutes to reflect on your emotions and thoughts. On Wednesdays, focus on staying hydrated and taking regular breaks to stretch.

Thursdays could involve socializing with friends or family in person or via video. On Fridays, brisk walks or hikes might be spent in nature to rejuvenate and connect with the outdoors. Saturdays could be reserved for practicing mindfulness and meditation exercises, while Sundays involve relaxing hobbies or activities that bring you joy, such as painting, reading, or cooking.

To promote quality sleep, follow a bedtime routine consistently each night, including turning off all screens an hour before your intended bedtime.

Allow for flexibility and customization, adjusting your daily self-care routines to align with your unique needs, preferences, and lifestyle.

By committing to a wellness plan that prioritizes self-care for the entirety of the month, you will build resilience, develop positive habits, and foster a deeper connection with yourself, ultimately enhancing your overall well-being.

Additional Bonus Tips

Health Awareness Month is in September. Health Awareness month is an important time to focus on promoting overall health & well-being. It provides an opportunity for nurses and individuals, organizations, and communities to come together and raise awareness about various health issues. Nurses, by participating in initiatives and events, we can educate ourselves about the importance of taking care of our health and mental wellness. September serves as a reminder to prioritize your well-being and make positive changes in our everyday lives.

Nurses, take time out to schedule your annual physical and health exams. Getting your annual Gynecologist, Mammogram, dental cleaning, and checkups. Men, get your Prostate exams done. Lab work and any other wellness checkups are vital to prevention and early detection of any disease.

Many nurses smoke and use the bathroom, just a reminder that hand washing before you give patient care is the first line of wellness. Believe it or not, I have asked nurses to wash their hands. If you see something wrong, it's your duty as a nurse to speak up and say something.

Reminder to all nurses, hand washing frequently is vital for preventing infections and contaminations. Promoting wellness and wearing protective equipment, including gloves appropriate for patient contact, is crucial. Also, following your institution's standards of care and policy and procedures is necessary.

Wear support hoses if standing for long periods. We, as nurses, do so much walking; it's important to wear good-fitting shoes that offer support. Loose-fitting uniforms that are comfortable. Hygiene care is vital to you, your colleagues, and your patients- bathe and use deodorant daily. Daily brushing teeth and dental care is a must.

Keeping your nails short and manicured neatly as most hospitals don't allow artificial nails where direct patient care. Taking care of yourself is the best nursing practice to give your patients the best care.

Lastly, here is a special prayer for nurses:

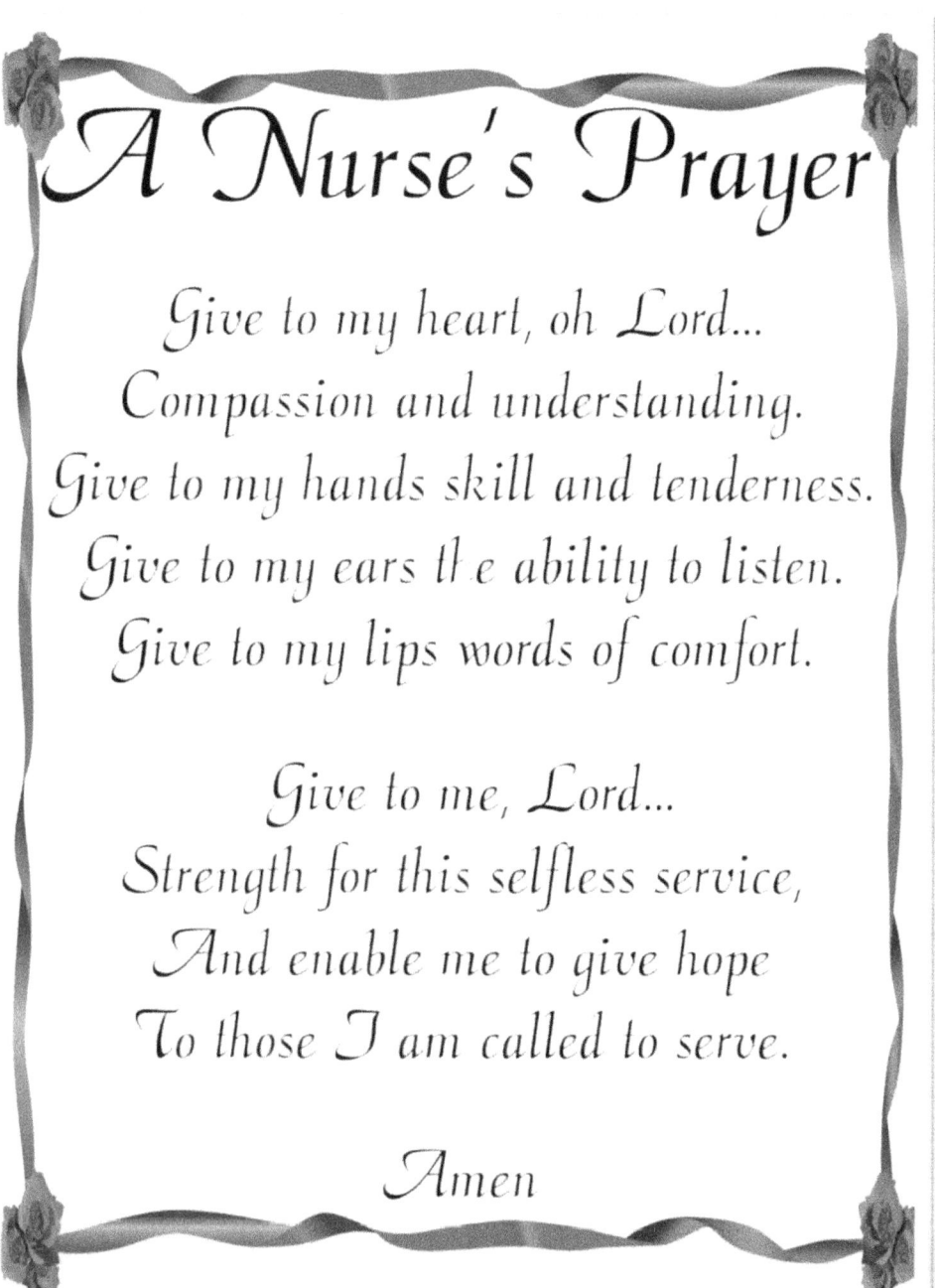

A Nurse's Prayer

Give to my heart, oh Lord...
Compassion and understanding.
Give to my hands skill and tenderness.
Give to my ears the ability to listen.
Give to my lips words of comfort.

Give to me, Lord...
Strength for this selfless service,
And enable me to give hope
To those I am called to serve.

Amen

"When you expect the best, you release a magnetic force in your mind which by a law of attraction tends to bring the best to you."

- Norman Vincent Peale

Notes

Notes

www.ingramcontent.com/pod-product-compliance
Lightning Source LLC
Chambersburg PA
CBHW070208230526
45471CB00002B/874